HYPERMOBILITY IN CHILDREN

A Guide For Parents And Caregivers

Ruth Peters

COPYRIGHT

Copyright © 2023 Ruth Peters

TABLE OF CONTENTS

INTRODUCTION

The Johnson family's life took an unexpected turn when their youngest daughter, Lily, was diagnosed with hypermobility syndrome at the age of seven. This diagnosis brought forth a set of challenges, but it also became an opportunity for the family to learn, grow, and support one another.

Lily's parents, Sarah and Mark, noticed that Lily's joints seemed more flexible than other children's. They initially brushed it off as a natural variation until Lily began complaining about joint pain and experiencing occasional dislocations during play. Concerned, they sought medical advice, leading to Lily's diagnosis of hypermobility syndrome.

Sarah and Mark were determined to understand Lily's condition and provide the best care. They began researching hypermobility, attending seminars, and connecting with online support groups. Armed with knowledge, they felt more equipped to navigate the challenges that lay ahead.

Lily's older siblings, Emma and Jake, became her biggest cheerleaders. They took the time to learn about hypermobility and helped Lily with her exercises and stretches. Sarah and Mark encouraged Lily to express her feelings and assured her that they were there to support her every step of the way.

As Lily entered school, Sarah and Mark collaborated closely with Lily's teachers and the school nurse. They created an Individualized Education Plan (IEP) that outlined Lily's needs and recommended accommodations. Lily's teachers provided alternatives during physical activities, and Lily's classmates learned about hypermobility to foster understanding and inclusivity.

Lily's parents enrolled her in physical therapy sessions to strengthen her muscles and improve her joint stability. Lily enjoyed the exercises and found camaraderie with other children in therapy. Her progress became a source of pride, and she began participating in activities she loved, like swimming and art.

Sarah and Mark made it a priority to promote positive body image in their home. They celebrated Lily's unique qualities, talents, and accomplishments. They encouraged Lily to focus on what her body could do rather than its appearance, fostering a healthy attitude toward herself.

The Johnson family found a supportive community of families dealing with hypermobility. They organized gatherings, sharing experiences and resources. Lily's journey became an inspiration for others, and she embraced her role as an advocate, speaking about hypermobility at school assemblies.

While Lily's hypermobility posed challenges, the Johnson family faced them with determination and unity. Lily's diagnosis became a catalyst for growth, empathy, and resilience. Through education, support, and open communication, the family learned that their bond was stronger than any challenge they encountered.

WHY THIS BOOK IS IMPORTANT FOR YOU

As parents and caregivers, your child's well-being is of paramount importance. One aspect that deserves your attention is hypermobility – a condition that involves increased joint flexibility beyond the normal range of motion. While some degree of flexibility is natural, excessive joint movement can have a significant impact on your child's physical health and overall development. Here's why it's crucial to understand hypermobility and its various types.

The Importance of Awareness

✓ Early Identification and Intervention: Recognizing hypermobility in its early stages empowers you to seek appropriate medical evaluation and intervention. Timely diagnosis can help manage any potential challenges and prevent complications from worsening over time.

✓ Understanding Your Child's Experience: Hypermobile children often experience joint pain, fatigue, and difficulties with physical activities. Understanding these challenges will enable you to provide the necessary support and accommodations to help them thrive.

✓ Preventing Overuse and Injury: Children with hypermobility are at a higher risk of joint injuries and overuse. By understanding their condition, you can guide them in safe physical activities and help prevent injuries.

Empowering Your Role

Armed with knowledge, you can become a stronger advocate for your child's needs. You'll be better equipped to communicate with medical professionals, educators, and other caregivers to ensure a supportive environment.

Understanding hypermobility allows you to provide holistic support that addresses both physical and emotional aspects. Your child might face challenges related to self-esteem, body image, and frustration. Your empathy and guidance can make a significant difference. Building Resilience: By learning about hypermobility and its types, you can guide your child towards building resilience and embracing their uniqueness. Teaching them how to navigate challenges positively can help them grow into confident individuals. By staying informed, you're equipping yourself to play an active role in helping your child lead a healthy and fulfilling life despite the challenges posed by hypermobility.

CHAPTER 1

HYPERMOBILITY UNVEILED

Hypermobility refers to an increased range of motion in the joints beyond what is considered normal. This flexibility occurs due to the structure of the connective tissues and ligaments surrounding the joints. While some degree of flexibility is natural and healthy, excessive joint movement can lead to various challenges and complications, especially in children.

Types of Hypermobility

Hypermobility can manifest in different ways and severity levels. There are two main categories of hypermobility:

1. Generalized Hypermobility: This type involves excessive joint flexibility throughout the body. It can affect multiple joints, such as the fingers, wrists, elbows, shoulders, hips, knees, and ankles. Generalized hypermobility is often hereditary and can be observed in certain genetic conditions.

2. Localized Hypermobility: In this type, only specific joints or joint groups exhibit increased flexibility. This could be due to various factors, such as injury, repeated overuse, or certain medical conditions affecting particular joints.

Benign Joint Hypermobility Syndrome (BJHS)

One common classification is the Benign Joint Hypermobility Syndrome (BJHS). This refers to a condition in which joint hypermobility is present without any underlying medical condition causing it. Individuals with BJHS may experience symptoms such as joint pain, fatigue, and joint instability, but these symptoms are not caused by a known inflammatory or connective tissue disorder.

Hypermobile Ehlers-Danlos Syndrome (hEDS)

Another well-known type of hypermobility is Hypermobile Ehlers-Danlos Syndrome (hEDS). This is a hereditary connective tissue disorder characterized by joint hypermobility, skin that is often soft and stretchy, and other symptoms like chronic pain and joint instability. hEDS can have a significant impact on a child's quality of life and requires careful management.

CAUSES AND RISK FACTORS

As a parent or caregiver, it's natural to be curious about the factors that contribute to your child's health and well-being. When it comes to hypermobility, it's important to understand the causes and risk factors that can play a role. By delving into these aspects, you can better navigate your child's journey and provide the appropriate support.

Causes of Hypermobility

✓ Genetics

In many cases, hypermobility has a genetic component. If you, your partner, or other family members have a history of joint flexibility, there's a possibility that your child might inherit this trait. Certain genetic conditions, such as Ehlers-Danlos syndrome, can also lead to hypermobility.

✓ Connective Tissue Structure

Hypermobility occurs when the connective tissues, ligaments, and collagen structures around the joints are more lax than usual. This can allow joints to move beyond their normal range of motion. The exact mechanisms behind this variation in connective tissue structure are still being studied.

Risk Factors for Hypermobility

✓ Gender and Age:

Hypermobility tends to be more common in females and children. As children grow, their connective tissues may become less flexible, and some hypermobility may naturally decrease with age.

✓ Family History:

If you have a family history of hypermobility or related conditions, your child might have an increased risk of developing hypermobility as well.

✓ Physical Activities:

Certain physical activities or sports that involve repetitive joint movements and stretching can contribute to hypermobility. While staying active is important, it's also crucial to strike a balance and provide proper guidance and supervision.

✓ Joint Injuries:

Injuries to joints, especially at a young age, can sometimes lead to increased joint flexibility. Joints that have been injured might develop greater mobility during the healing process.

✓ Hormonal Changes

Hormonal fluctuations, especially during puberty, can affect the elasticity of connective tissues and potentially contribute to hypermobility.

Learning about the causes and risk factors of hypermobility empowers you as a parent or caregiver. By staying informed, you can take proactive steps to ensure your child's comfort, health, and well-being. Working closely with healthcare professionals and fostering open communication will contribute to the best possible outcomes for your child's joint health and overall development.

RECOGNIZING HYPERMOBILITY IN CHILDREN

As parents and caregivers, your keen observation and understanding play a crucial role in ensuring the well-being of your child. Hypermobility can sometimes go unnoticed but has significant implications for a child's physical comfort and development. This section will help you recognize the signs of hypermobility in children

Understanding the Signs

✓ Unusual Joint Range of Motion:

Observe how your child moves their joints. Hypermobility can manifest as joints that extend, bend, or rotate more than expected. For example, you might notice your child's elbows or knees bending backward more than usual.

✓ Bendy Fingers and Thumbs:

Pay attention to your child's fingers and thumbs. Hypermobile children might have fingers that bend back at the knuckles, forming a shape similar to a "Z."

✓ Double-Jointedness:

While the term "double-jointed" isn't medically accurate, it's often used to describe hypermobility. If your child easily demonstrates movements that seem unusual or impossible for others, it could be a sign of hypermobility.

✓ Frequent Sprains or Dislocations:

Children with hypermobility might experience a higher frequency of joint sprains or dislocations due to their joints' increased flexibility.

✓ Joint Pain and Fatigue:

Complaints of joint pain, especially after physical activity or prolonged periods of standing or sitting, can be indicative of hypermobility.

✓ Flat Feet and High Arches:

Examine your child's feet. Hypermobile children might have flat feet or excessively high arches, which can affect their gait and posture.

Observing Daily Activities

✓ Difficulty with Fine Motor Skills:

If your child struggles with tasks that require fine motor skills, such as holding a pencil or buttoning a shirt, it could be due to hypermobility affecting their hand and finger joints.

✓ Fatigue During Activities:

If your child seems to tire quickly during physical activities or complains of discomfort, hypermobility might be a contributing factor.

If you notice any of the above signs or if you have concerns about your child's joint flexibility, it's important to consult a healthcare professional. A pediatrician, orthopedic specialist, or a rheumatologist can assess your child's joint flexibility, conduct necessary tests, and provide appropriate guidance.

Recognizing hypermobility in children requires attentive observation and awareness of the signs. By staying vigilant and seeking professional evaluation when needed, you can provide the appropriate care, support, and resources to help your child thrive and develop in a healthy and comfortable manner.

CHAPTER 2

IMPACT OF HYPERMOBILITY ON CHILDREN

Hypermobility affects children in different ways, depending on the severity and distribution of joint flexibility. While some children might experience only mild effects, others may face more pronounced challenges. It's important to recognize that the impact of hypermobility can extend beyond physical discomfort to affect emotional and social aspects of a child's life.

PHYSICAL CHALLENGES

As a parent or caregiver, understanding the physical impact of hypermobility on children is essential for providing the right care and support. Some of the physical challenges includes:

Joint Instability and Mobility Challenges

Hypermobility can lead to joint instability, making it difficult for children to maintain balance and coordination. This can impact everyday activities such as walking, running, and playing sports.

Pain and Discomfort

Children with hypermobility may experience pain and discomfort, especially after physical activities. Be attentive to your child's complaints of pain and provide appropriate rest and pain management strategies.

Risk of Injuries

The increased flexibility of hypermobile joints can make children more susceptible to injuries like sprains, strains, and dislocations.

Orthopedic Complications

In some cases, hypermobility can lead to orthopedic complications like scoliosis (curvature of the spine) or flat feet.

DEVELOPMENTAL IMPACT

As parents and caregivers, you play a crucial role in supporting your child's holistic development. Hypermobility can have significant effects on various developmental aspects of your child's life. Here are some of the developmental impact;

✓ Children with hypermobility might struggle with developing both gross and fine motor skills. These skills include activities such as running, jumping, climbing, writing, and manipulating small objects.

✓ Hypermobility can affect a child's balance and coordination due to joint instability.

✓ Children with hypermobility may find it challenging to participate in sports and active play.

EMOTIONAL AND SOCIAL IMPACT

As parents and caregivers, you are well aware of the intricate balance between your child's physical and emotional well-being. Hypermobility, can extend its effects beyond the physical realm, influencing your child's emotional and social experiences. Here are some emotional and social impact of hypermobility on children

✓ Children with hypermobility might struggle with body image concerns due to perceived physical differences.

✓ Hypermobile children may avoid participating in physical activities due to concerns about their flexibility or appearing different from their peers.

✓ Children who are different from their peers might face social isolation or even bullying.

CHAPTER 3

MEDICAL MANAGEMENT OF HYPERMOBILITY

As a parent or caregiver, you play a pivotal role in the health and well-being of your child. Hypermobility, requires careful medical management to ensure your child's comfort and development.

The medical management of hypermobility is centered on two main principles: pain management and joint support

PAIN MANAGEMENT

Pain is a common challenge faced by children with hypermobility due to the increased flexibility of their joints. Effective pain management is essential to ensure your child's comfort and quality of life. Here are various pain management strategies that can help alleviate discomfort and promote your child's well-being.

1. Physical Therapy

Physical therapy is a cornerstone of pain management for hypermobility. A skilled therapist can design exercises that focus on joint stability, muscle strengthening, and improving overall body mechanics. These exercises help reduce pain, enhance joint support, and promote proper movement patterns.

2. Gentle Stretching and Range-of-Motion Exercises

Incorporate gentle stretching and range-of-motion exercises into your child's routine. These exercises help maintain joint flexibility and prevent stiffness while minimizing the risk of overextension.

3. Joint-Protective Techniques

Teach your child joint-protective techniques, such as avoiding excessive joint movement or maintaining proper alignment during physical activities. These techniques can prevent strain and reduce the likelihood of pain.

4. Heat and Cold Therapy

Heat therapy, such as warm baths or heating pads, can help relax muscles and ease discomfort. Cold therapy, like ice packs, can reduce inflammation and numb painful areas.

5. Over-the-Counter Pain Medications

Consult with your child's healthcare professional before using over-the-counter pain medications. They might recommend suitable options to alleviate pain and inflammation, such as ibuprofen or acetaminophen.

6. Prescription Medications

For severe pain, a healthcare professional might prescribe pain medications. These should only be used under the guidance and supervision of a medical expert.

7. Assistive Devices and Medication

Assistive devices like braces or orthotics can provide support to hypermobile joints, reducing pain and improving stability during activities.

8. Ergonomic Considerations

Ensure that your child's environment, including furniture and workspaces, promotes good posture and minimizes strain on joints.

9. Rest and Recovery

Encourage your child to listen to their body and rest when needed. Adequate sleep and periods of rest can help manage pain and promote healing.

10. Mind-Body Techniques

Mindfulness, deep breathing, and relaxation techniques can help your child manage pain by reducing stress and promoting a sense of calm.

11. Hydration and Nutrition

Staying hydrated and consuming a balanced diet rich in anti-inflammatory foods can support joint health and alleviate pain.

12. Communication and Advocacy

Encourage your child to communicate openly about their pain and discomfort. Teach them how to advocate for their needs and seek help when required.

Pain management strategies for children with hypermobility require a combination of approaches. By implementing a holistic plan that includes physical therapy, lifestyle adjustments, and supportive measures, you can help your child experience relief from pain, improve their overall function, and enhance their quality of life.

NUTRITION

Proper nutrition is a cornerstone of supporting your child's overall health and well-being, especially when they have hypermobility. A balanced diet can help promote joint health, energy levels, and overall development. Here's a comprehensive guide to nurturing nutrition for children with hypermobility:

✓ Offer a variety of nutrient-dense foods, including whole grains, lean proteins, fruits, vegetables, and healthy fats. These foods provide essential vitamins, minerals, and antioxidants.

✓ Foods rich in omega-3 fatty acids, such as fatty fish (salmon, mackerel, sardines), flaxseeds, chia seeds, and walnuts, can help support joint health and reduce inflammation.

✓ Protein is essential for muscle growth and repair. Include lean sources of protein like poultry, fish, beans, lentils, eggs, and dairy products in your child's diet.

✓ Calcium and vitamin D are crucial for bone health. Include dairy products, fortified foods, leafy greens, and exposure to sunlight to support strong bones.

✓ Encourage your child to drink water throughout the day. Proper hydration supports joint lubrication and overall bodily functions.

✓ Reduce the consumption of processed foods high in added sugars, unhealthy fats, and artificial additives. These foods can contribute to inflammation and impact overall health.

✓ Opt for whole grains like brown rice, whole wheat, quinoa, and oats. These provide sustained energy and essential nutrients.

✓ Incorporate colorful fruits and vegetables rich in antioxidants. These foods can help reduce oxidative stress and inflammation in the body.

✓ Aim for balanced meals that include a combination of carbohydrates, proteins, and healthy fats. This balance supports sustained energy levels and overall well-being.

✓ Encourage your child to eat smaller, balanced meals throughout the day to maintain consistent energy levels and support their active lifestyle.

✓ Iron is important for energy production and overall health. Include iron-rich foods like lean meats, poultry, fish, beans, lentils, and fortified cereals.

✓ Teach your child about portion control to avoid overeating. Encourage them to listen to their body's hunger and fullness cues.

✓ Limit sugary snacks and beverages. Excess sugar can contribute to inflammation and impact overall health.

✓Consult a healthcare professional before considering omega-3 supplements. These can be beneficial for joint health, but individual needs vary.

✓Consider consulting a registered dietitian who specializes in pediatric nutrition. They can provide personalized guidance based on your child's dietary preferences and needs.

✓ Foster a positive attitude towards food. Teach your child to view food as nourishment and enjoy a variety of foods without guilt.

✓ Model healthy eating habits and positive attitudes toward nutrition. Children are more likely to adopt healthy behaviors when they see them practiced by adults.

✓ If your child has dietary restrictions, allergies, or sensitivities, find creative ways to include nutrient-rich alternatives that meet their needs.

✓ Consistency is key to reaping the benefits of a balanced diet. Encourage your child to make healthy food choices regularly.

By following these guidelines, you can provide children with hypermobility the essential nutrients needed to support joint health, energy levels, and overall growth. Tailor your approach to your child's preferences and needs, and always consult with healthcare professionals when making significant dietary changes.

CHAPTER 4

JOINT SUPPORT

Children with hypermobility often face challenges related to joint instability and increased risk of injury due to their flexible joints. Strengthening muscles plays a crucial role in providing joint support and reducing the likelihood of injuries.

Here are some examples of muscle strengthening exercises suitable for children with hypermobility. Remember to consult a healthcare professional before starting any exercise program, especially if your child has specific medical considerations. These exercises focus on promoting joint stability and overall muscle strength while minimizing the risk of joint injury:

1. **Planks**:

   - Have your child start in a push-up position with their elbows directly under their shoulders.

   - Keep the body in a straight line from head to heels, engaging the core muscles.

   - Hold the position for a few seconds and gradually increase the duration as their strength improves.

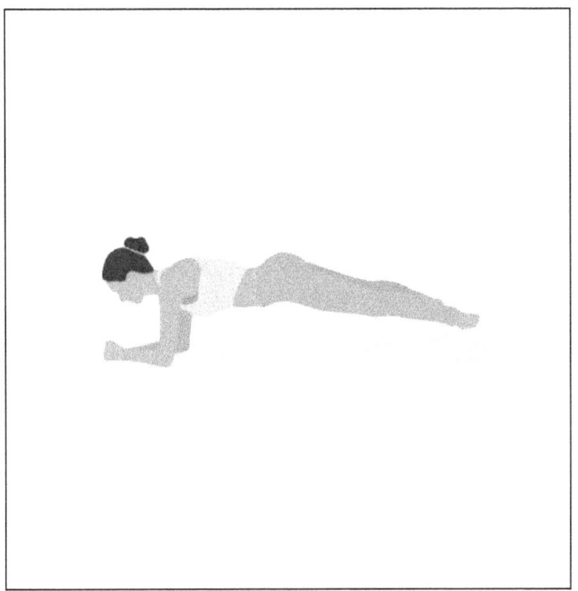

2. **Bridge Pose:**

- Have your child lie on their back with knees bent and feet flat on the floor.

- Instruct them to lift their hips off the ground, creating a straight line from shoulders to knees.

- Encourage them to squeeze their glutes and hold the position for a few seconds before lowering back down.

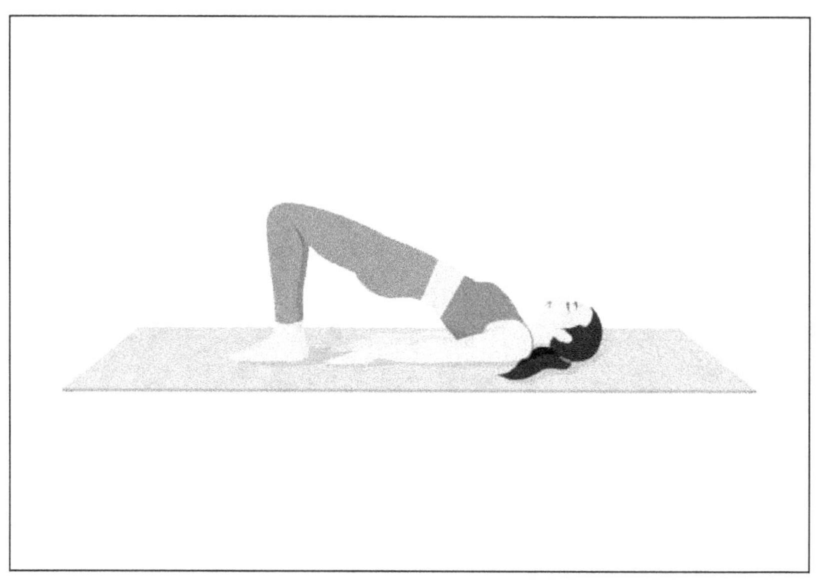

3. **Squats**:

  - Teach your child how to perform squats with proper form. Keep their feet hip-width apart, chest up, and knees aligned with the toes.

  - Have them lower their hips back and down as if sitting in a chair, then return to a standing position.

  - Start with bodyweight squats and gradually progress to holding a small weight if appropriate.

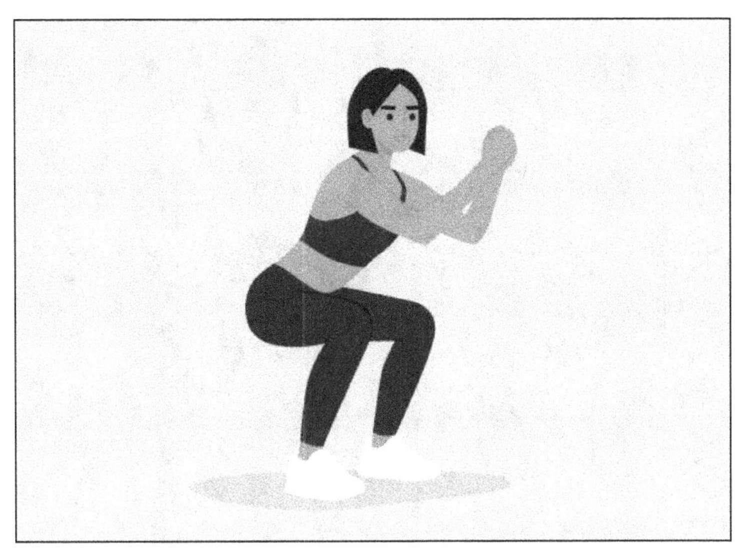

4. **Seated Leg Lifts:**

- Have your child sit on the edge of a sturdy chair with their back straight.

- Instruct them to lift one leg straight out in front of them while keeping the foot flexed.

- Lower the leg back down and repeat on the other side.

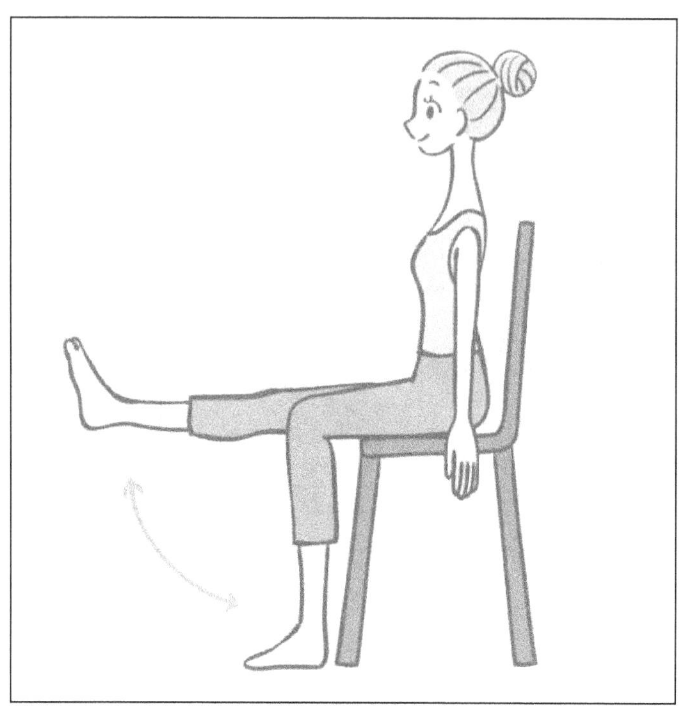

5. **Resistance Band Exercises**:

- Resistance bands can be used to add gentle resistance to exercises.

- Your child can perform exercises like bicep curls, tricep extensions, and seated rows using resistance bands.

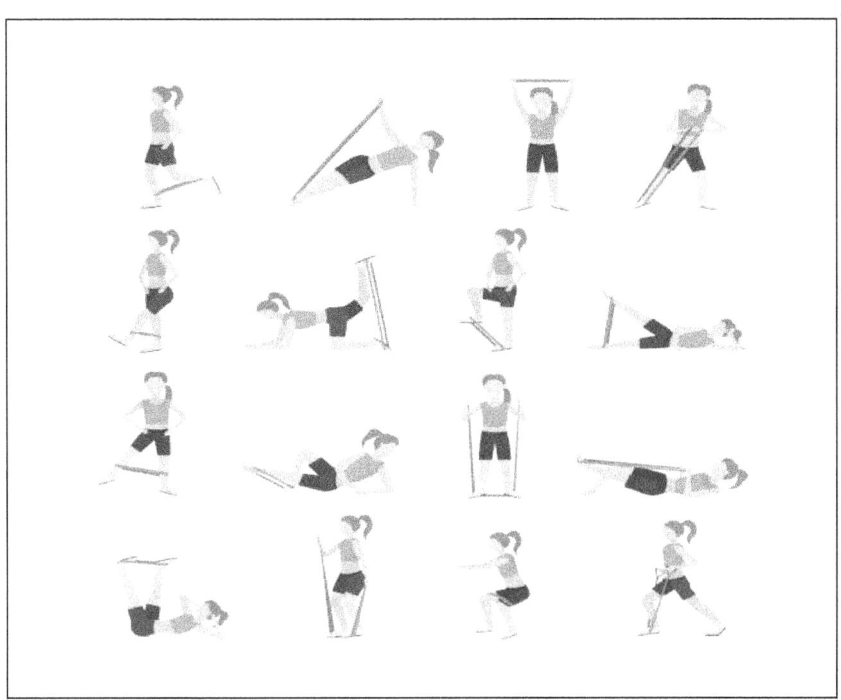

6. **Wall Push-Ups:**

 - Position your child facing a wall with arms extended, hands placed on the wall at shoulder height.

 - Instruct them to perform push-ups by bending their elbows and then pushing back up.

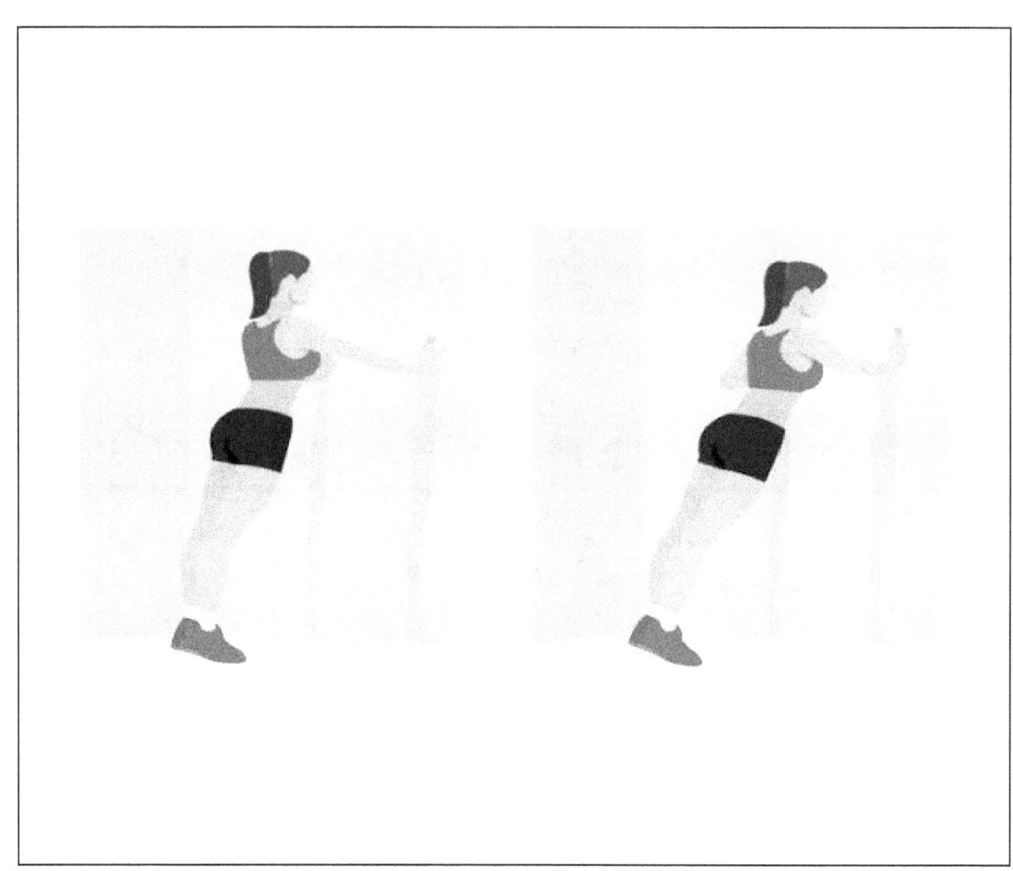

7. **Swimming**:

   - Swimming is an excellent full-body exercise that supports muscle strength and cardiovascular fitness without putting excessive stress on joints.

8. **Cycling**:

- Cycling on a stationary bike or a regular bicycle is a low-impact exercise that engages the leg muscles and improves cardiovascular health.

Tips for muscle strengthening exercises

When guiding children with hypermobility through muscle strengthening exercises, it's important to follow certain dos and don'ts to ensure their safety and optimize the effectiveness of the exercises. Here's a list of dos and don'ts to keep in mind:

Dos:

1. Before starting any exercise program, consult a healthcare professional, such as a pediatrician, orthopedic specialist, or physical therapist, to ensure that the chosen exercises are safe and appropriate for your child's condition.
2. Begin with low-intensity exercises and gradually progress in terms of intensity, duration, and complexity. This helps prevent overexertion and reduces the risk of injury.
3. Emphasize correct form and alignment during each exercise. Proper form reduces the risk of joint strain and supports effective muscle strengthening.
4. Encourage your child to engage their core muscles during exercises. A strong core provides stability and supports proper posture.

5. Incorporate exercises that target different muscle groups to ensure balanced muscle development and prevent muscle imbalances.
6. Advise your child to perform exercises with controlled movements. This helps prevent overextending joints and minimizes the risk of injury.
7. Depending on the exercise, provide appropriate support, such as using a stability ball, chair, or wall for balance if needed.
8. Include exercises that improve proprioception (awareness of body position) and balance. These exercises help enhance joint control and reduce the risk of falls.

Don'ts:

1. Avoid Overstretching: While flexibility exercises are important, avoid excessive stretching that might lead to joint hyperextension or strain.
2. Don't Push Through Pain: Instruct your child to stop any exercise if they experience pain. Pain should not be ignored or pushed through, as it can indicate potential joint damage.
3. Avoid High-Impact Exercises: High-impact exercises like jumping or running might increase the risk of joint injuries. Choose low-impact alternatives that provide cardiovascular benefits without excessive stress on joints.
4. Don't Rush Progression: Gradual progression is key to preventing injuries. Avoid rapidly increasing the intensity, duration, or complexity of exercises.

5. Avoid Poor Posture: Ensure your child maintains proper posture during exercises. Poor posture can strain muscles and joints.
6. Don't Neglect Rest and Recovery: Adequate rest and recovery time are essential for muscle repair and growth. Avoid overtraining.
7. Don't Compare to Others: Every child's abilities and limitations are unique. Avoid comparing your child's progress to that of others.
8. Avoid Unsupervised Workouts: Children with hypermobility should be supervised during exercises to ensure proper form and safety.
9. Don't Ignore Professional Advice: If a healthcare professional advises against specific exercises, follow their guidance.

By following these dos and don'ts, you can create a safe and effective muscle strengthening program for children with hypermobility. Always prioritize your child's safety, comfort, and well-being while helping them build strength and stability.

ASSISTIVE DEVICES

Assistive devices can play a significant role in supporting children with hypermobility, helping them manage their condition and engage in daily activities with greater ease and comfort. Here are some common assistive devices for children with hypermobility and how to use each:

1. **Orthopedic Shoes and Insoles**

Purpose: Orthopedic shoes and insoles provide proper support and stability to the feet, promoting proper alignment and reducing strain on the joints.

How to Use: Consult with a podiatrist or orthopedic specialist to determine the appropriate type of shoes or insoles for your child's needs. Ensure that the shoes fit well and provide adequate arch support. Insoles can be inserted into existing shoes to improve comfort and alignment.

2. Joint Supports and Braces

Purpose: Joint supports and braces provide additional stability to hypermobile joints, helping to prevent excessive movement and reduce the risk of injury.

How to Use: Consult a healthcare professional to determine the appropriate type of joint support or brace for your child's specific joints. Follow the instructions provided by the healthcare professional for proper fitting and usage.

3. Ergonomic Seating

Purpose: Ergonomic chairs and seating promote proper posture and alignment, reducing strain on the spine and supporting joint health.

How to Use: Choose chairs with adjustable features that allow your child to customize the seat height, backrest angle, and armrest height. Encourage your child to sit with their feet flat on the ground and their back against the chair's backrest.

4. Adaptive Writing Tools

Purpose: Adaptive writing tools with ergonomic grips or larger handles can help children with hypermobility hold writing utensils more comfortably and with improved control.

How to Use: Provide your child with adaptive pens, pencils, or grips that suit their needs. These tools can be used during writing and drawing activities to reduce strain on the fingers and wrist.

5. Stability Balls

Purpose: Stability balls provide a dynamic seating option that engages core muscles and promotes better posture and balance.

How to Use: Choose a stability ball with an appropriate size for your child's height. Encourage your child to use the ball as a seating option during activities such as reading or doing homework. Remind them to maintain proper posture while sitting on the ball.

6. Adaptive Utensils and Cutlery

Purpose: Adaptive utensils and cutlery feature modifications that make eating easier for children with limited grip strength or joint flexibility.

How to Use: Provide your child with adaptive utensils that have larger handles, ergonomic grips, or angled designs. These adaptations can help them hold utensils more comfortably during meals.

7. Mobility Aids (if necessary)

Purpose: Mobility aids such as crutches, canes, or walkers may be recommended in cases where joint instability affects walking.

How to Use: If prescribed by a healthcare professional, follow their guidance on how to use mobility aids safely and effectively. Ensure that the aids are adjusted to the appropriate height and that your child receives proper training on their usage.

Before introducing any assistive device, it's important to consult with healthcare professionals such as orthopedists, physical therapists, or occupational therapists. These professionals can provide personalized recommendations based on your child's specific needs and ensure that the devices are used correctly. Additionally, encourage your child to actively participate in the process and provide feedback on their comfort and experience with the assistive devices.

CHAPTER 5

PRACTICAL STRATEGIES FOR PARENTS

In this chapter, we will dive into how you can help your child overcome the impact of hypermobility. The developmental, social and emotional impact.

NAVIGATING THE DEVELOPMENTAL IMPACT

Parents and caregivers play a crucial role in helping children with hypermobility navigate the developmental challenges they may face. Here are some strategies to support your child's growth and development while addressing the impact of hypermobility:

✓ Educate yourself about hypermobility, its effects, and how it might impact your child's development. This knowledge will empower you to provide appropriate support.

✓ Foster open communication with your child about their condition. Explain hypermobility in an age-appropriate manner, addressing their questions and concerns.

✓ Focus on your child's strengths and achievements. Positive reinforcement can boost their self-esteem and motivation to overcome challenges.

✓ Encourage your child to develop independence and self-help skills. Provide guidance and support while allowing them to take on age-appropriate responsibilities.

✓ Work on fine motor skill development through activities like coloring, cutting, and using utensils. Provide tools that accommodate their needs, such as adaptive writing tools.

✓ Support your child in developing gross motor skills by engaging in activities like swimming, yoga, or dance. Focus on building strength, coordination, and balance.

✓ Consider enrolling your child in occupational or physical therapy sessions. Therapists can provide exercises and techniques tailored to their needs.

✓ Collaborate with teachers and school staff to ensure your child's needs are met. Discuss potential accommodations or modifications to support their learning and participation.

✓ Encourage your child to adapt and find creative solutions to challenges. Problem-solving skills are valuable for overcoming obstacles.

✓ Development is a journey that takes time. Be patient with your child's progress and provide ongoing support.

✓ Celebrate each step of your child's developmental journey. Whether it's a new skill learned or a milestone achieved, acknowledging their efforts boosts confidence.

By implementing these strategies, you can create a supportive and nurturing environment for your child. Remember that every child is unique, so tailor your approach to your child's individual needs, strengths, and challenges.

PROMOTING PHYSICAL ACTIVITY AND STRENGTH

Physical activity is crucial for the overall well-being of children with hypermobility. It can help strengthen muscles, improve joint stability, and enhance overall quality of life. Here are practical tips to promote physical activity and strength your child

✓ Before starting any physical activity program, consult a healthcare professional who specializes in hypermobility or pediatric orthopedics. They can provide tailored guidance based on your child's individual needs and limitations.

✓ Choose activities that are gentle on the joints, such as swimming, cycling, walking, yoga, and Pilates. These activities promote strength and flexibility without putting excessive stress on hypermobile joints.

✓ Prior to physical activity, encourage your child to warm up with gentle stretches and movements. Afterward, guide them through a cool-down routine to prevent stiffness and promote relaxation.

✓ Incorporate age-appropriate strengthening exercises that target major muscle groups. Consult a physical therapist or fitness professional to ensure proper form and safe progression.

✓ Engage your child in playful activities that involve movement, such as dancing, jumping on a trampoline with caution, and playing active games like tag.

✓ Incorporate balance exercises and activities that improve proprioception (awareness of body position), such as balancing on one leg or walking on uneven surfaces.

✓ Choose supportive and well-fitting footwear that provides stability during physical activities. Proper footwear can reduce the risk of joint strain.

✓ Teach your child the importance of pacing themselves during physical activities. Encourage them to take short rest breaks if they feel fatigued.

✓ Adjust the intensity and duration of activities based on your child's comfort level. Gradually increase as their strength and endurance improve.

✓ Supervise your child during physical activities to ensure they are performing exercises correctly and safely.

✓ If your child is interested, consider enrolling them in sports that are low-impact and offer skill development, such as swimming, martial arts, or gymnastics.

✓ Find activities your child enjoys and make physical activity enjoyable. Incorporate play, music, or family participation to make it a positive experience.

✓ Set achievable goals that align with your child's abilities and needs. Celebrate their progress, whether it's an increase in strength or improved endurance.

✓ Provide praise and positive reinforcement for their efforts and accomplishments. Encouragement boosts motivation and self-esteem.

✓ Engage in physical activities as a family. Outdoor walks, bike rides, or nature hikes can encourage physical movement while fostering family bonding.

✓ If your child is anxious about physical activity, create a supportive environment where they can express their concerns. Gradually introduce activities to build their confidence.

✓ Be willing to adapt activities to suit your child's needs. Modify exercises or choose alternatives if certain movements are uncomfortable.

✓ Celebrate even small achievements and efforts. Recognizing progress builds a positive attitude toward physical activity.

By following these practical tips, you can create a positive and supportive environment that encourages physical activity, strength development, and overall well-being in your child.

ADDRESSING SELF ESTEEM AND BODY IMAGE

Building self-esteem and fostering a positive body image is essential for the well-being of all children, including those with hypermobility. Here are practical tips to help you promote self-esteem and a healthy body image in your child

✓ Demonstrate self-acceptance and positive body image through your own actions and words. Children often learn by observing their parents' attitudes.

✓ Encourage your child to focus on their inner qualities, talents, and strengths rather than solely on physical appearance.

✓ Create an open and non-judgmental environment where your child feels comfortable discussing their feelings about their body.

✓ Teach your child that being healthy and active is more important than conforming to a specific appearance.

✓ Refrain from making negative comments about your own body or others' appearances. Negative body talk can influence a child's perception of their own body.

✓ Help your child critically analyze media messages and images that may promote unrealistic beauty standards. Discuss how images are often edited and do not reflect reality.

✓ Support your child in expressing themselves through their interests, hobbies, and passions, helping them develop a strong sense of identity beyond appearance.

✓ Help your child set achievable goals that are not solely based on appearance. Celebrate their accomplishments and efforts.

✓ Celebrate what makes your child unique. Encourage them to embrace their individuality and appreciate the diversity in others.

✓ Compliment your child on their kindness, perseverance, creativity, and other positive qualities unrelated to appearance.

✓ Teach your child to replace negative self-talk with positive affirmations. Help them develop a kind and encouraging inner dialogue.

✓ Discuss strategies for dealing with teasing or bullying related to appearance. Equip your child with tools to respond confidently.

✓ Encourage physical activity for the joy of movement and the sense of accomplishment it brings, rather than for changing appearance.

✓ Teach your child about self-care routines that help them feel good about themselves, such as proper hygiene, healthy eating, and adequate sleep.

✓ Help your child appreciate their body's abilities and the things it allows them to do, rather than focusing on its appearance.

✓ Support friendships with peers who value each other for who they are rather than how they look.

✓ Create a home environment where your child feels accepted and loved unconditionally, regardless of appearance.

✓ Encourage your child to focus on what they are grateful for in their lives, shifting their attention away from appearance-related concerns.

By implementing these practical tips, you can help your child develop a strong sense of self-esteem, a positive body image, and a healthy attitude towards self. Remember that building self-esteem is an ongoing process, and your consistent support and encouragement make a significant impact on your child's well-being.

NAVIGATING SCHOOL AND SOCIAL ENVIRONMENT

Navigating school and social settings can present unique challenges for children with hypermobility. By fostering open communication, providing education, and advocating for your child's needs, both parents and children can navigate these settings successfully. Here are practical tips to help you navigate school and social situations:

For Parents

✓ Inform teachers, school nurses, and other relevant staff about your child's hypermobility. Provide information on how it might impact their physical activities and any necessary accommodations.

✓ Work with the school to create an action plan that outlines your child's needs, potential challenges, and recommended accommodations. This plan can guide teachers in providing appropriate support.

✓ Maintain open communication with teachers and school staff. Discuss any changes in your child's condition and collaborate on adjustments as needed.

✓ If your child requires assistive devices or adaptations, ensure they are available and accessible at school. This might include ergonomic seating, adaptive writing tools, or joint supports.

✓ Teach your child social skills and strategies to navigate interactions with peers. Role-playing scenarios and practicing effective communication can boost their confidence.

✓ Encourage your child to communicate their needs and advocate for themselves when necessary. This skill is valuable for fostering independence.

For Children

✓ Understand your physical limitations and listen to your body. Don't push yourself too hard during physical activities.

✓ If you experience discomfort or pain, communicate with your teachers or supervisors. They can help you find alternative ways to participate.

✓ Engage in physical activities you enjoy and feel comfortable doing. Choose low-impact options that promote strength and flexibility.

✓ Pace yourself during physical activities and take breaks if needed. It's okay to rest when you feel fatigued.

✓ Connect with peers who appreciate you for who you are. Focus on building meaningful friendships that support your well-being.

✓ Educate your friends about hypermobility in a simple way. Help them understand your needs and limitations.

✓ Embrace your unique qualities and strengths. Confidence comes from knowing and valuing yourself.

✓ If you need assistance or accommodations, don't hesitate to ask for help. Teachers, school staff, and friends are there to support you.

✓ Prioritize self-care by getting enough sleep, eating nutritious foods, and managing stress. These practices contribute to your overall well-being.

✓ Focus on your achievements and what you can do, rather than what you can't. A positive attitude can help you overcome challenges.

By working together, parents and children can create a supportive and inclusive environment in school and social settings. With effective communication, education, and a positive outlook, children with hypermobility can thrive academically, socially, and emotionally.